Uncover Your Personality

Modified and modernized psychoanalytic theory made simple, understandable, and applicable.

Dr. Ryan YJ Chong

MBBS (Hons), MPM

Copyright © 2024 Dr. Ryan Yung Jie Chong

All rights reserved.

ISBN: 978-1-7635515-0-3

This book is dedicated to those who suffer and to those who are trying to alleviate suffering in any way that they can.

CONTENTS

	Acknowledgments	i
	Foreword	1
1	Inspirations	5
2	Personality Versus Temperament	11
3	Biological Determinism	17
4	Conscious Versus Unconscious	23
5	Substitute Personality	28
6	Social Feedback Mechanism	33
7	Conclusions	40
	Afterword	45

ACKNOWLEDGMENTS

This book is dedicated to the amazing staff at H&SCCT whom I have had the privilege to work closely with. I am deeply appreciative of your clinical support whilst I was busy fine-tuning aspects of this theory. I am also extremely grateful for your support in my personal development during the process.

Thank you to my friends. Whether it be peripheral via large groups or regular one-on-one meetings, I appreciate the support that you have given me whilst I uncover my personality.

Thank you to my mentors. If you have mentored me at any stage, you have made a significant contribution to where I stand currently. I hope that I will meet you again someday, but maybe in a different fashion, maybe as a peer instead of a student.

I must mention Tembie individually because she insists that she needs a mention. She does not get any royalties. Apologies. But it pays to ask.

Finally, thank you to my family. But they also had to ask to get a mention. Apologies.

FOREWORD

My practice in psychiatry as a trainee has given me the opportunity to help patients, for which I remain extremely grateful. In the process, I have had to interact with each of them on a personal level and I feel privileged to have joined some of them on a highly introspective journey of self-discovery. I similarly recall setbacks during my practice that I would wish to avoid, in the future, with a better understanding of human personality. Unfortunately, the human personality is not something that has been fully explained by my clinical experience or by any literature that I have read during my training in medicine and psychiatry. It remains a theoretical concept not yet proven by science. Yet, psychiatry currently regards some personalities as disordered despite a lack of scientific basis. I found this preconception simultaneously confronting and confusing. How can we decide if a personality is normal if we cannot even clearly define what a personality encompasses?

This question led me to wonder if human personality could ever be defined.

There were many theories that I perused but no

clear answers. I still felt that I had an obligation to, at least, try to find an answer, if not for myself and my clinical practice, then, at least for the sake of my patients and their mental wellbeing. Thus, I embarked on a personal journey to try to find out more about what exactly encompasses a human personality. In doing so, by reviewing the multiple concepts that have been put forth by previous experts in the field of psychoanalysis, I did manage to find individual parts of a greater concept that appeared so nebulous and complex that I had to write it down. When I finally managed to scrouge together a concept that worked in combination with my knowledge and experience, it ended up being such a hefty idea that it would fill a book. It was a working theory of personality in full, but it was so complex that it would take ages to categorically explain it to anyone. Let alone patients in distress.

I decided that I should try to publish this theory in the form of a book anyway, despite the complexity, because I strongly believe that mental health is the most important aspect of health. With personality as a core component that is yet to be fully explained or understood, surely, then, personality should be an area that society should explore and develop as a concept with regards to mental wellbeing. But with such a complex concept, the theory had to be made as streamlined and as accessible as possible, so that it could be communicated easily. A refined and simplified version of the theory had to be developed. This newer, modified, and streamlined theory of personality coalesced. This theory largely relies on the individual delving into their unconscious mind and bringing everything they find towards their conscious mind, and thus I rely on the concept of "uncovering" as an easily understandable analogy to summarize the key point of the theory. Thus, the book promises that it will help you "uncover" your personality as a means of achieving greater understanding of your personality. Hopefully, this also translates to improved mental wellbeing. I can only hope that my goal has been achieved through what has been written within this book. In any case, if this theory is deemed incorrect by the opinion of others, I still hope that this book can, at least, serve as a basis for deeper discussion about the true definition of personality.

Hopefully, you now understand my motivation behind the creation of this theory. There are also a few caveats to note before we launch into the "uncovering" of the human personality. I need to make it very clear that the contents of this book are completely theoretical. I may be wrong on many points. Personality is complex, ever changing and by no means is this book definitive when discussing personality. I publish this book mainly as I aim to provide a basis for discussion about personality and what it could be. As this book is completely theoretical, I do not cite any specific references and it is not meant to be an academic manuscript. Instead, I acknowledge the many contributions from historical figures in the field of psychoanalysis, whom I refer to within this theory, and I ask that you review their psychoanalytic theories separately so that you may arrive at your own conclusion. Also, as I appreciate the complexity of trying to capture the essence of human personality using words, I will try to summarize my theoretical musings and condense important ideas into simpler terms at the end of each chapter. Hopefully, this will allow you to continue reading on even if some concepts do not directly appeal to you.

Finally, I will discuss challenging topics which may directly affect your understanding of your own identity and personality.

Please be aware of your mental state and seek professional help when necessary.

1 INSPIRATIONS

This theory was inspired by the collective body of work from various experts who have been recognized for their significant individual contributions to the field of psychoanalysis. I specifically draw inspiration from Sigmund Freud, Carl Jung, Anna Freud, Melanie Klein, and John B. Calhoun. I will systematically list and discuss exactly where and how their ideas are utilized to uncover your personality.

Be reassured that it is not necessary for you to completely understand the ideas that are discussed within this chapter. I draw reference solely because I wish to recognize the phenomenal existing body of work that has graciously allowed for this theory to coalesce.

I, firstly, completely rely on the previously known concept of biological determinism, also sometimes termed genetic determinism. Biological determinism is the idea that human behaviour is completely dependent on physical factors. This will be evident throughout the theory as a key component of personality.

To begin naming specific expert psychoanalysts, we must, obviously, first discuss concepts from the founder of psychoanalysis himself, Sigmund Freud. Sigmund Freud was a famous neurologist and psychoanalyst. He is renowned for various psychoanalytic concepts, one being his theory of psychosexual development. He has already developed a theory of personality that should be familiar to all. His concept of the psyche is broken down into three main components - the id, the ego, and the superego. Whilst I deeply respect his contribution to psychoanalysis, by virtue of attempting to develop a different theory of personality, my view diverges somewhat. Thus, I must explain where any deviation occurs. I do not refer to his theory of psychosexual development as I do not find that any developmental state can be clearly applied towards human personality. I also do not explore his concept of the psyche as defined by the id, the ego, and the superego, as I seek to provide a different perspective altogether with the conclusion of this theory. Of course, I may just be completely wrong. It could be theoretically possible that his concepts co-exist in conjunction with this theory. However, I will have to, for now, focus on describing the current theory and defer this conversation to a later stage.

This theory frequently refers to his topographic theory of the unconscious, which is better known as the iceberg theory. This is the concept that the human mind consists of two parts. It consists of the conscious mind being the visible part of the iceberg, floating above the sea, whereas the unconscious mind is the submerged and thus invisible part of the iceberg. Both parts exist simultaneously, but only one is visible from the surface.

This theory also frequently refers to the Freudian slip. Classically, Freudian slips are seemingly trivial errors in speech which are believed to occur as the unconscious mind blends into consciousness. Sigmund Freud expanded the meaning of the Freudian slip to include other behavioural errors such as miscommunication and tardy behaviour.

I will later discuss the combination of the Freudian slip and the topographic iceberg theory of the unconscious as central tenets to this theory of personality.

Next, Anna Freud was a psychoanalyst and the daughter of Sigmund Freud. She is well known for her contribution to child psychoanalysis. Anna Freud expanded on her father's idea of ego defence mechanisms by defining specific immature ego defences. More importantly, she considered ego defences as automatic and sometimes unconscious mechanisms. I refer to her idea that immature ego defences are automatic and unconscious mechanisms when discussing how the human personality may react whilst it is being uncovered. I utilize dualities to consider the negative aspects of immature ego defences when discussing this theory.

What are dualities? To understand dualities, we must look towards the work of Carl Jung, another famous psychoanalyst. He is still compared to the likes of Sigmund Freud even to this day. He is known for many ideas, examples being the collective unconscious and archetypes, for instance. However, I solely draw inspiration from his idea of dualities. The idea is best explained by examining Carl Jung's dualities of the shadow and the persona, and the anima and the animus. The central idea of dualities is that one aspect cannot exist without the other aspect. If one aspect is observable, the other aspect must exist as well. According to dualities, the human persona must be backed up by a shadow, and every human carries within themselves the forces of the anima and the animus regardless of their gender. I find that dualities are strongly related to Sigmund Freud's topographic iceberg theory, where the conscious mind and the unconscious mind simultaneously co-exist within the human mind as a single entity. I refer to dualities frequently to consider aspects of personality that are hidden from view and thus need to be uncovered.

I note that Carl Jung has created his own theory of the unconscious mind. He divides it into two parts, namely the collective unconscious and the individual unconscious. He has defined the collective unconscious as the parts of the human brain, which all humans possess, that contribute to the unconscious process. In contrast, the personal unconscious arises from the individual life experiences that cannot be consciously processed by the human mind for various reasons. Again, whilst I deeply respect his contribution to psychoanalysis, by virtue of attempting to develop a different theory on personality, my view diverges somewhat.

Thus, I must explain where any deviation occurs. This theory incorporates biological determinism as a key concept. We will conceptualize the human brain as being, potentially, fully unconscious. This is an important deviation from Carl Jung's theory of the collective unconscious as part of the brain. This theory notes that it could be the whole brain that is collectively unconscious. Thus, this theory diverges.

Furthermore, I will discuss my concept of a society-based communal unconscious dynamic, coined the "social feedback mechanism", in a later part of the book. This has no resemblance to how Carl Jung has defined his concept of the collective unconscious as an individual part of the individual human brain. Again, I may just be completely wrong. Again, it could be theoretically possible that his concepts co-exist in conjunction with this theory. However, I will have to, for now, focus on describing the current theory and defer this conversation to a later stage.

Following on, Melanie Klein was a psychoanalyst who is well known for her ideas regarding object relations theory. In this theory, infants are thought to internally separate the good and bad aspects of their parental figures, literally seeing these parts as separate objects which can only be unified through consistent parental attachment. I draw inspiration from this theory to consider that an individual's personality could also be fluid because it is internally compartmentalized and thus not yet successfully integrated. It is an important idea to keep in mind.

However, I do not explicitly refer to this concept when discussing the theory.

Finally, John B. Calhoun was a behaviouralist famous for his "rat utopia" experiments which demonstrated that, in overpopulated animal models, complete provision of material needs still led to behavioural regression on a societal level that was termed the "behavioural sink". As part of this theory, I do consider how the "behavioural sink" phenomenon might occur when personality is not well understood by society.

Thus, I have clearly specified the creators and ideas that are, in my opinion, crucial to keep in mind whilst we uncover the secrets of the human personality. These ideas already exist within the current body of literature, though. Some might ask, then, what exactly do I bring to the table? Where is my input towards this theory? Most people forget or were not aware that Sigmund Freud was a qualified neurologist. I am not a qualified neurologist. However, I do have medical knowledge and clinical experience in the field of psychiatry. I wish to utilize my knowledge and experience to interpret an immense body of information left behind by the previous leaders in psychoanalysis. I aim to provide a modern perspective that should spark some renewed discussion. I do, also, conceptualize new ideas, that, when combined with the ideas previously noted, form a robust view of human personality. In doing so, my hope is that this book could provide a novel, holistic, and yet streamlined, concept of personality.

2 PERSONALITY VERSUS TEMPERAMENT

To begin in earnest, we need to try to define personality. Personality is currently a nebulous concept. In defining personality, I have considered the long-debated question of nature versus nurture. This question is important because the idea has always been that nature was determined and thus unmodifiable, whereas nurture was variable and thus modifiable. Sometimes, life goes completely perfectly for a person, and yet they turn out to be behaviourally disordered as defined by society. Sometimes, life goes completely awry for a person, and yet they turn out to be completely behaviourally normal as defined by society. How can this observable difference be reconciled? Perhaps the answer lies in the duality of temperament and personality.

What is temperament? The temperament of a child was always thought to be a factor that was determined in the womb. Perhaps the current explanation for the above-mentioned contradiction in outcomes is that the individual's temperament was simply incompatible, or conversely too compatible, with social norms. No amount of personality modification would have made any difference. The good person was always going to be good, regardless of what bad things happen to them that could shape their behaviour towards acting against social norms. Conversely, the bad person could never be good, no matter how many good things happen to them that could shape their behaviour towards acting in a socially acceptable manner. It seems that temperament as a concept can be seen as fixed, unmodifiable, and static. Thus, temperament is thought to be the "nature" aspect of observable human behaviour for the purposes of this theory.

But, of course, this theory discusses personality. In direct contrast to temperament, the personality of the child, and later adult, is thought to be a process that is continuous and modifiable. It is thought that personality can change, for better or worse, throughout the lifespan of a human being. This was undoubtably the case in my clinical practice where I personally observed how personalities can change on a day-to-day basis. It is also true that I have directly experienced personality change during significant life events, as noted by my own introspective process. Thus, it seems that personality can be static at times, but is also fluid, variable and modifiable at other times. Personality, then, must be the "nurture" aspect of observable human behaviour.

And, indeed, psychiatry as a movement seeks to directly address and modify personality that is deemed disordered by social standards. You will recall, at this point, that I am concerned about modifying personality when it has not been clearly defined. How do we define personality then?

An important distinction between temperament and personality then arises for consideration. Temperament as a concept can be seen as fixed, unmodifiable, and static. Meanwhile, personality as a concept can be static at times, but is also fluid, variable and modifiable at other times. Could it be that temperament is far less complex whilst personality is extremely complex? Maybe this is why no one has really been able to clearly identify or define personality. Is it too large of a concept to comprehend for one person? Maybe we need to rely on the fact that personality is likely to be more complex. Perhaps we need to be as broad as possible in the definition. Let us use the idea that personality is the "nurture" aspect of observable human behaviour. What can be nurtured in a person? I will admit that it took a long time to come up with this definition. Going as broadly as possible, I believe that it can be defined by a combination of an individual's spoken words, measured actions, memories, life experience and emotional state, made more difficult to externally quantify due to some aspects being unconscious and others conscious to the individual.

These are all aspects of human behaviour. However, you will note that I have started to include psychoanalytic concepts to explain why personality could be static at times, yet variable, fluid, and modifiable at other times. My answer to my own question about the definition of personality spawned the ideas that are yet to be discussed.

I promised earlier in the book that a medical perspective would be included in this theory. How, then, does personality and temperament relate to the human as an organism? Medical knowledge posits that the seat of any human consciousness must be situated within the human brain. Indeed, even the controversial philosophical thought experiment of the brain in a vat still recognizes that a human brain must be involved with regards to human consciousness. Personality and temperament must then involve the human brain but in different aspects. Consider, then, that within the human genetic makeup there lies a DNA blueprint for the genesis of human neural tissue. Perhaps within the DNA blueprint lies the concept of temperament, the unmodifiable aspects of a human mind. With this idea it stands to reason that the personality, or the modifiable component of a human mind, lies within the structure of the neural tissue itself. Interestingly, we do know that neuroplasticity and neurogenesis are processes that can occur within the human brain to change brain structure and function. Perhaps this explains why personality can be static but also variable. It would depend on whether neuroplasticity, or neurogenesis, or both, are active processes. And what, then, does the neural tissue hold? It is known that speech centres, motor centres, memory centres and emotional centres are defined parts of the human brain. Perhaps, then, personality is the complex combination of an individual's neural connectome.

Perhaps an individual's personality is approximately 1,200 grams of neural tissue, or approximately 85 billion neurons. This potentially equates personality to be the externally observable and internally recognizable aspects of a human having a human brain. Does this idea fit in with the previously mentioned definition of personality? Both are of similar complexity. I see similarities between the two definitions, which is why I have incorporated psychoanalytic concepts into my discussion about human personality as a definitive necessity. I am fortunate enough to have both medical and psychoanalytic perspectives of personality, and thus I continue to explore both approaches simultaneously throughout the rest of the book.

But, not to get too far ahead of ourselves, let us consider the implications of this definition of personality as the gestalt of human neural tissue. Well, this definition could mean that your personality is a unique combination of every single internal perception that you experience, and every single externally observable behaviour that you exhibit. As an example, what you might eat for breakfast tomorrow could be just as important, in terms of your personality, as how you might feel when you propose marriage to your life partner. Surely, then, it is impossible for a single person to be completely aware of every single aspect of their brain. You would have to be aware of every single neural connection within your brain. Perhaps it is possible, but only with concerted effort expended consistently over time.

But, as we have noted previously, personality is fluid, variable and modifiable. What happens then when we are aware of some connections but unaware of others? To begin answering this important question, we proceed then to the psychoanalytic aspect of this theory which will be discussed from the next chapter onwards. As you will see, personality is extremely complex. As promised, I will do my best to simplify these concepts.

However, first, the promised streamlined summary of this chapter.

In summary, it is important to make a distinction between temperament and personality. Temperament likely arises from the genetic DNA blueprint for the creation of human neural tissue. Personality is far more complex than temperament. Personality likely encompasses the entirety of the individual's neural tissue, approximately 85 billion neurons, each with their connections to other neurons that contributes to the internal workings and external observable behaviour of an individual's personality, whether they are aware or unaware of each connection.

Let us move on.

3 BIOLOGICAL DETERMINISM

To understand how awareness, or consciousness, is a key factor in personality, we must firstly revisit the concept of biological determinism. What is determinism? Determinism, in general, is the concept that the outcome of a specified system will always be the same. Run a deterministic computer program a million times and the outcome will be the same. Biological determinism, then, is the idea that human behaviour is completely dependent on physical factors. If the concept of biological determinism is valid, it would imply that everything that you did, felt, remembered, or said was predetermined because you have a human brain. Your life would be one continuous Freudian slip, all because you were born with a functional human brain.

I start the theory by proposing that biological determinism is a key component of personality. Basically, because you have a brain, and you rely on it to function, I believe that you could theoretically function even if you were completely unaware of any neural connection in your brain. I recognize that it is a confronting concept to believe that the human being is a machine that could potentially function in a completely unconscious state. This completely goes against the concept of free will. Even so, I had to wonder if biological determinism could be linked to personality. I had to confront this disturbing concept many times throughout my clinical practice when observing chronic patterns of seemingly automatic human behaviour. A good example of seemingly automatic human behaviour that should be known to all is disassociation. There were no clear answers to explain why I had observed disassociation in my patients. There was no clear explanation of how a personality could be involved when a patient experienced disassociation, despite the very clear fact that it had originated from the human being before my very eyes. Thus, to start getting answers, I first combined the concept of biological determinism with Sigmund Freud's theory of the Freudian slip to arrive at the first psychoanalytic aspect of this theory.

As a thought exercise, consider a Freudian slip where you did something without even realizing that it occurred. It is important to remember that the Freudian slip is a human behaviour. After all, Sigmund Freud was trying to explain what he had observed in his human patients when he conceptualized the idea of the Freudian slip. An example could be that you so unconsciously dread seeing your doctor to get your blood test results, and so you turn up late to your appointment unintentionally. You completed an action without realizing it. How could you have completed that action without realizing it? How could a human being behave in an unconscious manner if free will exists? Well, anatomy currently contends that the human being is controlled by the human brain. If the human being completed a specific behaviour, regardless of whether it was aware or not, the neural connection must have existed within the human's brain, prior to when the human completed the specified behaviour. The first aspect of this theory, then, is that every behaviour, whether conscious or not, must exist within the human neural circuitry before said behaviour is carried out.

Thus, based on the concept of the Freudian slip, the idea of biological determinism is valid. You always had the neuron in your brain that was going to cause you to behave in a certain manner. Indeed, functional MRI scans can contemporaneously show you exactly which parts of your brain are in use when you perform a specific task. This was the first iteration of the theory. However, note that, at this stage, personality should be completely fixed in nature because it is completely predetermined. Thus, this first aspect of the theory is incomplete because it cannot explain the variability of personality as previously defined. Clearly, a piece is missing.

It is confronting yet interesting, then, to combine the first iteration of this theory again with Sigmund Freud's iceberg theory of the conscious and the unconscious. I first thought that the human individual was always going to behave in that manner because it was predetermined by the neural connection that was present in the brain that allowed it to occur. However, a distinctive human experience could lie in whether the human being was aware or unaware of what was always going to happen. The Freudian slip is not a trivial error, but instead a predetermined outcome, based on the first iteration of this theory, so then, which part of personality is variable? Is it not, then, that the only variable portion of personality is whether the human being was aware or unaware that said outcome was going to occur?

The second iteration of this theory, then, was that you always had the neuron in your brain, you were biologically determined to act that way, like a machine fulfilling its programming, and the variable aspect of observable personality then lies in whether you were acting consciously or unconsciously. This theory fits because it allows for a human brain to be a machine on the inside whilst appearing variable and fluid on the outside. In terms of personality, this theory importantly allows for personality to be a variable construct within the fixed framework of biological determinism, but only through Sigmund Freud's topographic iceberg theory of the unconscious.

At this point, you would appreciate that the theory is getting complicated. I must pause and reiterate that everything discussed so far is purely theoretical. It could be completely wrong. If anything, this theory should, at least, provide an appreciation of just how complex personality as a construct could be.

Let us continue now because an important point must be noted. If acting unconsciously, you made a Freudian slip, as it has been previously defined, and you would not be aware of it at the time. There is not much to discuss by default. What happens, then, if you were acting consciously and understood that your brain controlled your actions completely, but you continued to act in the same manner anyway? You would be conscious, and you would have given in to biological determinism. It is uncomfortable to contend that we could be following preset courses of action, but in this consideration, a duality is revealed. Maybe you could change your preset course of action if you were aware of said preset course of action. Maybe you could be aware of how your brain automatically makes you do things, feel things, and say things, and it is only then that you could choose to behave differently. Maybe, you could defeat biological determinism by uncovering your personality.

This is the proposed solution to the problem that the theory raises. But, before we move on, let us summarize. Generalizing on a neurobiological basis, this theory contends that the human being can assume control of all its predetermined actions only if said actions are drawn to consciousness. You must be completely aware of how you are behaving so that you can fully understand how you could modify your predetermined actions.

In simpler terms, as your brain controls everything, your brain holds your personality. This theory contends that, by default, you would unconsciously act in the exact same way every single time you replayed your life. Not to despair, because maybe there is a way to assume control if you were aware of what was going on in your brain, and thus, uncover your personality.

4 CONSCIOUS VERSUS UNCONSCIOUS

It has been raised that you would need to uncover your personality to effectively modify your predetermined actions. Let us talk about the process of uncovering your personality by implementing further psychoanalytic theories. Immature ego defence mechanisms have been described as automatic by Anna Freud. What are they and where do they lie in the human brain? These immature defence mechanisms are thought to be innate, and it is believed that humans tend to regress away from mature defence mechanisms towards immature defence mechanisms as, well, a defence mechanism to safeguard your sanity. An example of this could be that you like to exercise to relieve stress, but when stress overwhelms you, you may feel the need to yell indiscriminately as a method to vent your anger, instead of relying on exercise as you did previously. One might note that this example demonstrates regression from sublimation as a mature defence mechanism towards acting out as an immature defence mechanism. Medically, I believe that immature defence mechanisms are likely primitive neural connections that persist, likely from a young age, to protect us from catastrophic personality destruction. One would appreciate that this is a duality. A fragile personality construct will be shattered by the slightest insult, and the strongest personality construct could still be shattered by an overwhelmingly destructive insult. I bring up immature defence mechanisms because I believe that they help us conceptualize a difficulty that could arise when trying to uncover your personality.

Let us start by reverting to the iceberg theory, where most of the iceberg is submerged and a small portion is visible from the surface. By extension, if you consider that the brain is sitting in the same situation encased within your skull, where some neural connections are apparent to you whilst others are not, what is the outcome when you raise the iceberg out of the sea? What is the outcome when you raise the brain out of the unconscious? By allowing the individual to be fully conscious of their 85 billion neurons, the main change is not in the conscious elements that were already visible from the surface. Instead, the change is in the unconscious elements that were previously submerged and invisible, but now uncovered and apparent to the individual. What does the individual uncover? How does the individual change now that it has to consider the full 85 billion neurons contained within its brain, as opposed to a simplified existence where it had to consider far less than 85 billion neurons?

I started to wonder about what you would find

when you started sifting through your neurons. Multiple ideas came to mind but the one that stuck was developed by combining the second iteration of the theory with Anna Freud's theory that immature ego defence mechanisms are automatic. In the context of biological determinism, immature ego defence mechanisms must begin as unconscious aspects of personality if they are automatic, which, as defined by Anna Freud, they are. They must be something that you will find below the surface. They must be something that you must uncover. If you lift the iceberg out of the sea, what do you find? Do you not find automatic immature ego defence mechanisms? What are the implications?

Considering the implication of uncovering these immature defence mechanisms, I wondered about how the duality of conscious and unconscious might apply to immature defence mechanisms as well. When you consider the presence of these defence mechanisms, are you not, then, aware of their existence and function? Are you not, then, more aware of your predetermined behaviour? A duality could exist. Sure, these defence mechanisms are meant to protect you from serious psychological harm. What happens if the nature of immature "ego offence" mechanisms is that they also automatically cause the human mind to feel uncomfortable, causing the human mind to avoid confronting thoughts, thereby lowering the iceberg back into the sea of the unconscious and preventing the human being from uncovering its own personality? The implication that arises here is that you could try to improve your awareness of your behaviour and thus uncover your personality, but in a similar fashion, there may exist biologically determined aspects of your brain that push you away from achieving full consciousness of your personality.

At this point, I have already noted many times that personality is a complex and variable concept. The presence of immature "ego offence" mechanisms would make the concept of personality even more complex because you now also need to contend with an in-built mechanism that actively opposes the act of uncovering your personality in the first place. This idea adds even more variability to the concept of personality, as now, the iceberg is constantly in a state of flux, slowly and automatically sinking back down whilst the human mind tries to raise it out of the ocean of the unconscious. Interestingly, it is at this point where I believe that the theory is finally fully developed. This is because the theory is so complex and variable that it might just explain why human personality is so complex and variable. It is finally a theory that is coherent with observable reality.

In which case, a question arises. The iceberg is always in flux and is potentially being dragged down by defence/offence mechanisms. Your brain potentially has an in-built mechanism that opposes your efforts to uncover your personality. Will there ever be a steady state where you could finally be free of this struggle? Is it even possible to fully uncover your personality?

This question is a crucial question that is essential to answer if we are to arrive at the conclusion of this book. I believe that this is not just achievable; it is the very definition of human self-determinism. It is the very definition of free will. However, I must, first, discuss factors that exist outside of the biologically determined personality. These factors possess duality in that they could be severe hinderances towards consciousness. Conversely, when addressed correctly, these factors could also provide a conduit towards improving consciousness of your personality. When addressed correctly, these factors could hold the key to your survival against the struggle that occurs in the process of uncovering your personality.

In summary, you could be a machine with a preset outcome. You may not have control over what you do by default. It could be theoretically possible to assume full control if you take the time to carefully look at your actions, your words, your emotions, and your memories, and in the process, uncover your personality. However, there may be factors within the machine itself that prevent you from assuming full control, and there will be a struggle associated with this conflict.

5 SUBSTITUTE PERSONALITY

So far, we have discussed the potential internal workings of personality. An aspect that has not been discussed is the external observable behaviour which I have previously listed as a core component of personality. Thus, it must be addressed by the theory. Which externally observable behaviours, then, are likely to be unconscious? My clinical experience as a medical professional immediately drew me to consider the role of external coping mechanisms, whether they be functional or destructive.

For the purposes of this discussion, coping mechanisms are regular and frequent actions that individuals undertake to deal with discomfort. It is important to consider coping mechanisms because the individual engages in these external coping mechanisms via their actions. Thus, engagement with the coping mechanism must arise from the brain if the theory is true. Examples of functional and socially acceptable coping mechanisms include exercise, meditation, and distraction. What then are destructive coping mechanisms? There are too many to list and these could be destabilizing for the individual whilst reading this book. I do, however, need to raise an example for the purposes of explaining this aspect of the theory. Thus, I believe that a common and somewhat socially acceptable coping mechanism, that could be safely raised as an example, is substance misuse.

A substance taken as a coping mechanism, by default, occurs because the individual expects that it will always work the same way and they will always get the same experience each time they use the substance. You will note that this pattern of behaviour is termed "misuse" and not "use". Dualities arise again. As a behaviour, the expectation is that substance misuse leads to a predetermined outcome. We have noted that any engagement with the coping mechanism must arise from the brain. How interesting, then, that an external stimulus can replicate the automatic and biologically determined process that is already present in the individual's neural tissue. What is even more interesting to consider is how the personality could be drawn to access this external stimulus repeatedly. What does this say about the inner workings of the human brain? Does it seek out external replications of internal processes? Is this an automatic process as well? I posit that the individual was always going to be attracted to coping via a specific substance if it replicated biologically determined aspects within the brain. It follows then, that substance misuse as a coping mechanism becomes an external biologically determined influence that could replace or enhance the internal biologically determined outcome of the individual's personality.

The classic pervasive example is alcohol use. Alcohol is classified as a depressant and is known to alleviate social anxiety when appropriately consumed. However, if you consumed alcohol frequently and did not understand why, one would consider that there was a specific anxiety component to your consistent consumption of alcohol. A deeper consideration would be that, as consistent substance misuse is a behaviour, your behaviour was predetermined, and you were always going to be vulnerable towards misusing that substance. Why, then, is the human individual using external coping mechanisms to replicate what was already present and predetermined internally? Perhaps this is also a biologically determined aspect of personality in general.

Bringing it back to a general discussion about coping mechanisms, there must be an aspect of the coping mechanism that is consistently experienced by the individual when the mechanism is repeatedly accessed. The internal workings of the unconscious human brain must be replicated externally, and thus the individual is, then, unconsciously drawn to utilizing this coping mechanism repeatedly. How interesting that the chosen language itself reflects the automatic nature of coping via a mechanism. Does this explain addiction?

How then, can this problematic aspect of personality be addressed? Using what was discussed in the previous chapters, an answer becomes apparent. Again, consciousness is the first step, and recognizing dualities is the second. Does the external coping mechanism exist only externally? Well, based on dualities, both internal and external aspects must exist simultaneously.

For the coping mechanism, there must be the substituted personality aspect. For the external coping mechanism, there must be an internal coping mechanism that lays dormant.

This is a powerful idea as it implies that there is a direct transcranial relationship between human personality and external coping mechanisms. What, then, are the implications of the presence of external coping mechanisms?

Regarding substance misuse, being conscious of your substance use pattern and the type of substances that you use frequently to cope can allow you to relinquish these substitute personality aspects in favour of developing your awareness of your own biologically determined personality. In doing so, you can uncover your personality instead of unconsciously drowning your personality in substances that replace the predetermined functions of your neural tissue. This is a salient point, with regards to comorbid substance misuse, which I have seen often in my clinical experience. Substance misuse can become a positive experience with the possibility of recovery and healing, but only if it is interpreted correctly by the operator as a positive experience.

By extension, this concept means that the use of any coping mechanism, whether it is deemed as socially acceptable or not, could still serve as a hindrance to uncovering your personality. This is because a personality usually accesses coping mechanisms via unconscious means. By uncovering your coping mechanisms, I imagine that the goal is to first convert them from automatic mechanisms to deliberate and conscious acts of self-care. You would still use them to cope at times, but at least you would be aware of it. This buys you time to perform effective introspection, allowing you to uncover parts of your personality. Later, you could remove the mechanism completely and cope with distress by utilizing novel, uncovered aspects of your personality, such as the hidden internal coping mechanism that you were covering up.

As if personality was not complicated enough already, this discussion regarding external coping mechanisms reveals another missing consideration. It reveals that we have not discussed how a personality might unconsciously interact with its external environment in general, and vice-versa if dualities are to be considered. Again, this must be considered so that the theory is made applicable to reality.

But first, the summary. In summary, you are disadvantaged if you avoid working on yourself and rely on external coping mechanisms, even if you can guarantee that these coping mechanisms can be available to you forever. You cannot uncover your personality until you accept the function of these external coping mechanisms in a conscious manner and work towards reducing your reliance on them.

6 SOCIAL FEEDBACK MECHANISM

This chapter starts somewhat differently. It starts with a review of the analogy of the iceberg floating in the sea of the unconscious. So far, the analogy has already been modified to include a rising iceberg and a sinking iceberg. I tried to extend the iceberg analogy to incorporate external coping mechanisms. It may not have been too successful as it is now a complicated analogy. But I seek your opinion regardless. It goes like this. I imagined that when you access coping mechanisms unconsciously, you unwittingly find a hand to push the iceberg further down into the sea of the unconscious. You could change this firstly by being aware of the presence of the hand. Thereafter, by using it to raise the iceberg out of the sea. Eventually, you will also have to remove the hand that you found unconsciously.

I appreciate that this makes the analogy clunky and complicated. It is better to just stick with the analogy that raising the iceberg is akin to uncovering your personality. Why do I bring it up then? I bring it up because it helped me consider if the iceberg could float above the sea naturally once it was raised and the hand was removed. In doing so, it sparked two considerations that arise from everything else that has been discussed previously.

Firstly, how could you achieve consciousness and uncover your personality in a vacuum, if some aspects are unconscious and must be accessed by a roundabout external system of coping mechanisms?

Secondly, how could the iceberg stay out of the water without the individual intervening against automatic immature defence/offence mechanisms that lower it back down automatically?

If personality was not complex enough, there remains the final aspect of the theory to round off before we conclude. The discussion so far has assumed that an individual biologically determined personality functioned in a vacuum. This is completely unrealistic. The personality of an individual exists within a swathe of separate personalities, all individually at variable levels of consciousness with regards to biological determinism. Yes, complexity and variability increase even further, but we must address this point to make the theory realistic and applicable.

Revisiting the considerations above, perhaps then, the most important aspect of society is that individuals were supposed to encourage elevation of unconscious processes towards consciousness on each other's behalf. This would cover both points that were raised as above. You would need other people around to observe your behaviour externally, so that they can redirect these aspects towards the correct internal channels to achieve effective introspection. If other people helped you keep your iceberg out of the sea for you, you would not have to intervene as often. You would not need to rely on coping mechanisms as they have been defined in the last chapter. You could assist other people with their personality whilst they assist you with yours, almost as a communal and personality-based symbiotic relationship. The result is communal reduction in external coping mechanism use whilst everyone gets to uncover their personality. Perhaps this is why society exists? An internal "social feedback mechanism" that exists to replace external coping mechanisms is beneficial for everyone, and thus humans congregate?

You would note, then, that there may be a conflict of interest that arises for individuals who are predominantly conscious of their behaviour. It is very difficult to move from unconsciousness towards consciousness if isolated from human contact. Such an individual must possess a metacognitive meta-neuron within the brain intrinsically if it were to self-self-actualize. Expecting default metacognition would probably be an extremely high expectation to ask of any individual. Ironically, individuals who operate unconsciously may also affect the level of consciousness within society if they predominate. Thus, it becomes more difficult for consciousness to increase communally when everyone engages in unconscious and automatic behaviour. This potentially ends as a "slippery slope" which results in self-perpetuating societal moral decline, perhaps linked to the concept of John Calhoun's overpopulated utopian "behavioural sink". Ideally, there would be internal ego strength within those who are conscious, but even then, these conscious individuals may be outnumbered, having to dedicate their time towards solving other pressing matters in society. These individuals may not have the time to help others keep their icebergs out of their seas. The outcome here is that society trends towards automatic and unconscious behaviour. Less and less people, over time, uncover their personalities. Thus, a conflict of interest arises as predominantly conscious individuals may not benefit from interacting with too many predominantly unconscious individuals.

Perhaps, then, the "social feedback mechanism" is necessary for society to allow individuals to uncover their personalities? What a duality. If this "social feedback mechanism" was not present, perhaps, then, there exists a role for external substitute personality structures to be utilized to positively move individuals, on a communal level, towards consciousness? Perhaps both substitute personality structures and the "social feedback mechanism" must first be created by the individuals within that specific societal structure? Perhaps that is why external media devices such as books exist?

Before moving on with this discussion, you will note that I have similarly devised the "social feedback mechanism" as a mechanism. I have done so because, in my mind, the "social feedback mechanism" acts by replicating externally what is present internally, akin to coping mechanisms as previously discussed. It could be an unconscious process that makes individuals gravitate towards each other. I imagine that this is because like would attract like. An unconscious individual would want to interact with another unconscious individual as it mutually externally replicates the individual's automatic and internal neural processes, in a sort of symbiotic relationship that results in mutual roundabout uncovering of individual personality. Thus, on a mass scale, a productive society is born via the "social feedback mechanism". How interesting that this could potentially be an unconscious and biologically determined process. How interesting that this could also be a part of the personality waiting to be uncovered. Perhaps the opposite of the "social feedback mechanism" is loneliness?

But let us return to the discussion. Again, a duality can be considered regarding external media devices and the "social feedback mechanism". Whilst the individual may desire to achieve consciousness, it may not be possible to achieve full conciousness of personality unless the societal construct provides a feasible environment for this to occur. If not via external means, consciousness will have to occur via internal means. But how is this even possible when the personality tends towards unconscious and automatic function? This perspective is troubling because it implies that individuals within a society with an unconducive environment must first act unconsciously to confront their internal demons, and thereafter cooperate to become aware of their personality. This implies that a period of social strife will first occur so that individuals can generate the required external societal construct that then allows them to uncover their personalities. External conflict will have to precede internal conflict. What is important, then, is that this period of strife is clearly defined as a constructive experience. Unfortunately, the deadly combination of communal unconscious dynamic and "behavioural sink" phenomenon could create a feedback loop, maliciously altering the trajectory of positive strife towards negative conflict, basically reinforcing the "behavioural sink" outcome as a function of socially pervasive and communally unconscious personality.

This is not an easy concept to internalize. It could also be wrong. However, it is a necessary discussion to consider when trying to uncover your personality, because you will be met with conflict in the process of uncovering your personality if the conditions within society are not conducive to introspection. Examples of barriers to introspection could include economic inequality, discrimination, or even political interference. Of course, solutions to these problems are not within the scope of this book.

One would also note that this concept could explain why the rate of mental illness is rising across the world, with depression projected to be a worldwide leading cause of disability. Perhaps societies in general are no longer conducive to introspection. This would result in increased automatic and unconscious behaviour, meaning less and less of the population can access the "social feedback mechanism". With reduced access to the "social feedback mechanism", uncovering personality becomes difficult and the individual reverts to the perpetual struggle against immature ego defence/offence mechanisms. The individual must also rely on external coping mechanisms instead of relying on other people via the "social feedback mechanism". This time, however, a solution to this problem is within the scope of this book. The solution lies within the scope of any deliberately fashioned external media device that encourages people to increase their awareness of their personality. Hmmm.

We are almost done. In summary, you will need to interact with external influences within a conducive social environment to fully uncover your personality. This may be other people, but it could also be human-created external media such as books. You may face difficulties when uncovering your personality due to problems in society. This is troubling and will likely lead to some form of conflict, and it is important that said conflict is civil to prevent a societal "behavioural sink" from occurring. I will refrain from commenting on how to fix problems in society as they are not within the scope of this book.

7 CONCLUSIONS

Let us recall the question, so that we can conclude this theory by answering the question in full.

To reiterate the question, I asked if there will ever exist a steady state where you could finally be free of the struggle between your conscious and unconscious mind. I asked if we could ever fully uncover our personalities.

Let us try to summarize how you could finally defeat biological determinism. Let us try to free ourselves from automatic behaviour. In doing so, we can finally understand and uncover our personalities.

This theory summarizes that, as an unconscious human being, you were always going to follow the same predetermined course of action if you played your life out a million times. This is due to your brain, and thus your personality, being biologically predetermined by default. This theory began by using and combining various psychoanalytic theories to consider the distinctive human experience that lies in whether the human being is aware or unaware of what was always going to happen. Due to the dynamic between the conscious and unconscious mind, any control over your predetermined course of action could occur only through a sequence of events.

Firstly, you would have to be in a social setting conducive to introspection. This is because an unconscious mind will have to begin any interpretation of the internal world via external means. This could be through interactions with other people, or it could be through interactions with human-created media. If this was not available, you would likely face internal and external conflict when trying to create a conducive setting. You would have to surmount such conflict.

You would then have to start gaining awareness of your actions, words, emotional state, and memories simultaneously. Some of these could be observable only by others and not yourself, and so you would have to take any advice from others with a positive viewpoint. This step could also involve you confronting the deepest aspects of yourself and accessing these aspects continuously, hopefully with an active awareness of any discomfort that is elicited in conjunction. Thus, the warning at the start of the book.

You may start to rely on coping mechanisms in the process of experiencing discomfort. You would then have to consciously appreciate and actively remove external coping mechanisms such as substance misuse. This is because these coping mechanisms can serve as an avenue towards self-discovery, but they will also eventually impede your ability to complete introspection.

You would then have to grow your consciousness

of your internal world and your external behaviour. Doing so would allow you to explore and uncover every aspect of your personality. Your progress must be consistently maintained because your brain has an in-built defence mechanism that, unfortunately, also acts against conciousness. Once you lose your awareness of your predetermined personality, you have lost control, and you tend to revert towards automatic behaviour due to the in-built defence/offence mechanism.

If you succeeded, you would finally defeat biological determinism and fully uncover your personality. I imagine that this is a beautiful cognitive state where human consciousness aligns completely with the fatalistic imperative that was always biologically determined. What would such a state even look like or feel like? I imagine that your words would completely correlate with your actions. You would know everything about yourself. You would have explored every single aspect of your internal world. You would be conscious of every single behaviour that you have previously completed, and maybe even some behaviours that you are yet to complete. You could be completely aware of how you were going to live your life, prior to the actuality of living out your life. I imagine that you would feel calm, fulfilled, and satisfied.

The final duality exists in an ironic fashion. Fully uncovering your personality could give you the freedom to explore endless possibilities. Having full knowledge of everything that you were, everything that you are, and everything that you will be, ironically, allows you to change your initially predetermined course of action. One might consider this phenomenon a beautiful combination of permanent identity formation and self-actualization.

To end the theory, finally, I believe that the alignment of full human consciousness and the biologically deterministic imperative allows for permanent identity formation and self-actualization. Personality, then, is the in-between state that occurs when a partially conscious human being grapples with the remaining unconscious elements of their brain. Personality is inherently unstable, which is why personality is so variable and complex. Identity is the outcome when the iceberg is completely raised out of the sea of the unconscious and the personality is fully uncovered. Self-actualization is the outcome when the knowledge of the fully uncovered human personality finally allows an individual to determine their actions against the biological imperative.

Thus, we reach the end of this theory. Hopefully, I have been successful in my pursuit of an answer. Hopefully, a medical perspective has allowed for the creation of a novel, modern, and modified psychoanalytic theory that holistically addresses the manifold complexities of personality within the human individual in a fashion that is as simplified, streamlined, and applicable as possible.

Notably, I recognize that some aspects of this theoretical perspective are not new. For instance, personality as an unstable intermediary step towards identity may not be a new concept. Self-actualization is also a concept that has previously been noted by others, most notably psychologist Abraham Maslow in his hierarchy of needs. In fact, some discussions within this book regarding societal problems are probably reflected by the hierarchy of needs required to achieve self-actualization according to Maslow.

However, I think it is very interesting that we arrive at a similar conclusion using a completely novel combination of psychoanalytic theory and modern medical perspective. I am hopeful, then, that this lends credence to the validity of this theory of personality. I would also not be surprised if this theory is only another piece of the extremely complex puzzle that is the human personality.

AFTERWORD

Clearly, my intention in writing and publishing this book is to elicit healthy debate and personal introspection. I have probably also sought to develop my own version of a "social feedback mechanism" in the form of an external media device. Perhaps this is my conscious or unconscious method of uncovering my own personality. I am glad if it motivates you to choose your own unique method of uncovering your personality as well.

I end the book with a collection of unsorted thoughts that came about whilst I was writing this book. They are currently unanswered in my mind, and so I raise them in the hopes of finding answers someday.

Firstly, this theory has significant implications for people who believe in free will as a given. It explains that, technically, a person could function in a completely unconscious state. People may not have free will by default. My theory implies that free will has to be achieved via a combination of social and psychological factors that will allow a person to perform deep introspection. Significant effort is required, and the individual must be willing to commit to this effort, perhaps even unconsciously as a biologically determined feature. What then of culpability defences in legal cases? How does this change your opinion regarding the individual and their responsibility for their human behaviour?

What new opinions may then be formed about societies that prioritize conflict and war? Are they simply avoiding introspection on a mass scale? What then of societies that completely devote themselves to consumption of external media? Again, is this avoidance of introspection on a mass scale? These are the tough questions about society that arise if this theory is valid.

What about temperament? We have discussed that temperament is quite different to personality. Perhaps the truth lies in duality. Perhaps the concept of temperament is simply a misnomer that describes the fixed and biologically determined aspect of personality that we could never consciously process until it was pointed out to us via external means. Epigenetics supports this idea as well, as it turns out that DNA can be modified by environmental stimulus at a basal level that is difficult to conceptualize. Does temperament even exist, then? I think that it must because personality exists. But perhaps temperament is complex, static at times, yet variable at other times, because of how temperament and personality exist as dual concepts.

On a slightly easier note, I also wonder about a point I made earlier. I wonder if there ever was, or ever will exist an individual with a meta-neuron that allowed for automatic metacognition, so that the individual could achieve full control over a biologically determined brain without any external help. This human theoretically would be fully conscious and would have uncovered their identity by default. It would completely invalidate the unconscious elements of this theory. One would wonder if this would even be a desirable existence. Will this person ever need to socialize?

I also wonder about the stages of brain growth that occur within the development of the child. Perhaps this is why child psychoanalysis has always been an interesting topic. As the brain tissue, and thus, by my theory, personality, develops during physical growth, maybe children and young adults were not subject to the same problems of biological determinism because their brain was not of fixed nature. Perhaps this is the so-called innocence of childhood, where the mind is flexible and free. Is it possible, then, that my theory only applies to adults whose brain has fully developed, thus "solidifying", becoming less modifiable in structure? Continuing in the vein of child psychoanalysis, what then of attachment theory, another famous theory created by John Bowlby? How does attachment theory correlate with this theory of personality in the child? I refrain from commenting because these two theories, in my mind, could be separate theories altogether. It could be that the growth of the human brain in childhood lends towards attachment theory, after which the outcome in the adult brain lends more towards personality and identity. Or, maybe, attachment occurs during the child's internal exploration of their personality via the external foils of their parents? Perhaps there is a link between attachment theory and the "social feedback mechanism"?

Finally, I wonder if personality testing is valid in two dimensions. Firstly, it could be valid in trying to categorically cover every single aspect of personality, and thus, map the human brain from a subjective standpoint whilst viewing from the outside inwards. This makes it an incomplete external media device that is in development as an attempt to enact the "social feedback mechanism". Perhaps we should also consider the value of simply having a person interact with their own personality via the test, which would then cause them to introspect and thus increase their consciousness of their personality. Maybe this is why any interaction with personality tests are always about the first answer that comes to your mind. I believe that it would be important to have the second aspect clearly stated as an objective of any personality test if this theory is true.

Perhaps, one day, a complete psychometric test will finally be able to encompass all aspects of personality. However, this theory implies that such a test would be extremely large and complex. Perhaps such a test would have to be individualized based on the unique known life history of the person taking the test, just to make it less cumbersome to administer. Perhaps a pre-test interview will be required for the test to be tailored to the profile of the person. Does this reduce its validity?

As a final note, I would like to thank you for reading past the conclusion of the book. Please recall that all external conflict must remain civil and that you should seek professional help if any internal conflict becomes unbearable. I remind you now, because, based on this theory, the only way to break free from a biologically determined brain is to be aware and to take control over it. And thus, the only way to break free from a biologically determined life is to fully uncover the unconscious aspects of your personality.

ABOUT THE AUTHOR

Dr. Ryan YJ Chong was born in Singapore. His middle name "Yung Jie" directly translates to "forever outstanding" in Mandarin, and thus he's known from birth that tall poppy syndrome is real. He moved to study medicine at Monash University in Victoria, Australia.

He now calls Australia home, at least for the time being. He is glad that helping others is part of his job description. As a trainee in psychiatry, he is grateful that he has been given the opportunity to publish his ideas about mental health.

He has a Bachelor of Medicine and Bachelor of Surgery (Honours) from Monash University, and a Master of Psychiatry from The University of Melbourne.

www.ingramcontent.com/pod-product-compliance
Lightning Source LLC
Chambersburg PA
CBHW071727020426
42333CB00017B/2429